Step by Step Mediterranean Diet Recipe Book 2021

Ultimate Step by Step Mediterranean Diet Recipe Book for Learn Healthy Eating Habits and Lose Weight!

Jim Smith

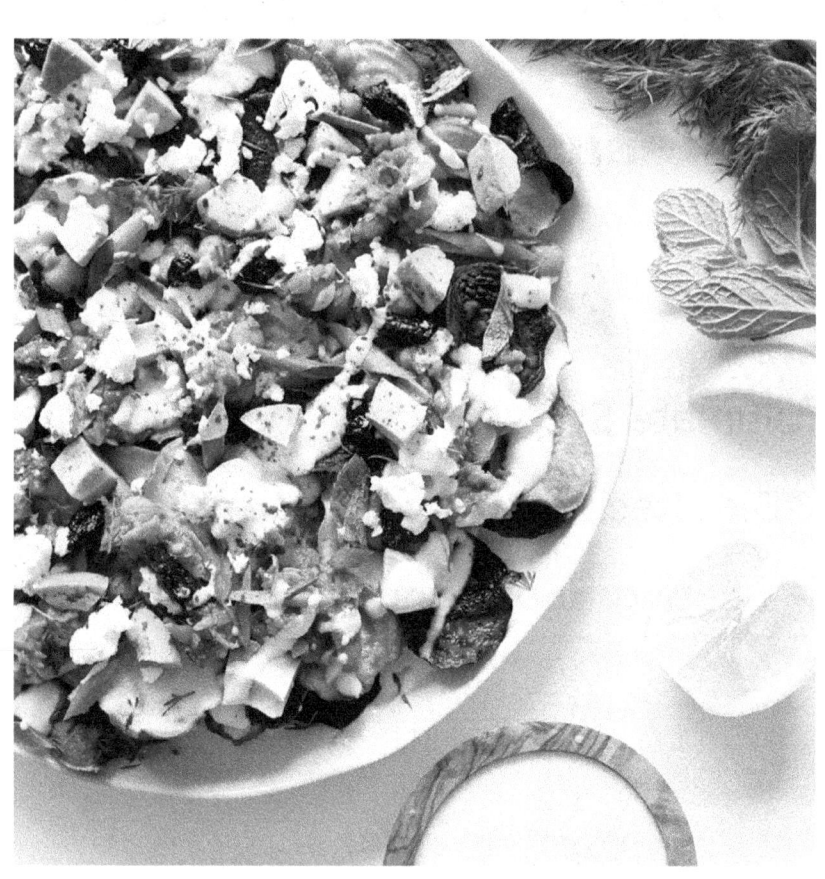

Table of Contents

INTRODUCTION — 10
- Crunchy Chickpeas — 15
- Stuffed Dates — 17
- Almond Gazpacho — 18
- Turkey Chowder — 21

PASTA AND COUSCOUS — 23
- Spaghetti Carbonara — 23
- Tagliatelle Pasta — 26
- Pasta "Verochka" — 29
- Pasta e Patate — 31
- Pasta with Fresh Tomatoes — 34
- Spaghetti Carbonara With Chicken — 36
- Carbonara With Fettuccine — 39
- Fast Spaghetti Carbonara — 41
- Pasta with Greens — 43
- Harvest Pasta — 46
- Pollo Mediterranean — 49
- Pasta Fagioli Soup — 52
- Pasta al Mediterraneo — 55
- Tomato Basil Penne Pasta — 57
- Whole Wheat Pasta Toss — 59
- Quick Mediterranean Pasta — 61
- Mediterranean Fish and Pasta Stew — 63
- Parsley Pesto Paste — 65
- Potato in Tomato Paste — 67
- Hummus — 69
- Hollandaise Sauce — 71
- Creamy Tahini Dip — 72
- Basil Lime Dip — 74
- Cilantro Dip — 75
- Tahini Sauce — 77
- Arugula Salsa — 78

RICE AND GRAINS — 80

Fragrant Basmati Rice	80
Cranberry Rice	82
Italian Style Wild Rice	83
Brown Rice Saute	84
Pesto Rice	86
Rice Salad	87
Rice Meatballs	88
Mediterranean Paella	89
Fast Chicken Rice	91
Rice Jambalaya	92
Jasmine Rice with Scallions	94
Cremini Mushrooms Pilaf	95
Vegetable Rice	97
Tomato Rice	98
Rice with Grilled Tomatoes	99
Rice and Meat Salad	100
Rice Bowl	101
Zucchini Rice	102
Rice Soup	104
Rice with Prunes	106
Rice and Fish Cakes	108
CONCLUSION	**111**

© Copyright 2021 by Jim Smith- All rights reserved.

The following Book is reproduced below with the goal of providing information that is as accurate and reliable as possible. Regardless, purchasing this Book can be seen as consent to the fact that both the publisher and the author of this book are in no way experts on the topics discussed within and that any recommendations or suggestions that are made herein are for entertainment purposes only. Professionals should be consulted as needed prior to undertaking any of the action endorsed herein.

This declaration is deemed fair and valid by both the American Bar Association and the Committee of Publishers Association and is legally binding throughout the United States.

Furthermore, the transmission, duplication, or reproduction of any of the following work including specific information will be considered an illegal act irrespective of if it is done electronically or in print. This extends to creating a secondary or tertiary copy of the work or a recorded copy and is only allowed with the express written consent from the Publisher. All additional right reserved.

The information in the following pages is broadly considered a truthful and accurate account of facts and as such, any inattention, use, or misuse of the information in question by the reader will render any resulting actions solely under their purview. There are no scenarios in which the publisher or the original author of this work can be in any fashion deemed liable for any hardship or damages that may befall them after undertaking information described herein.

Additionally, the information in the following pages is intended only for informational purposes and should thus be thought of as universal. As befitting its nature, it is presented without assurance regarding its prolonged validity or interim quality. Trademarks that are mentioned are done without written consent and can in no way be considered an endorsement from the trademark holder.

INTRODUCTION

The Mediterranean eating regimen is a way of life. It's a method of eating so as to carry on with a full and solid life. When following along these lines of eating you'll get in shape, yet you'll likewise reinforce your heart and give your body all the best possible supplements important to carry on with a long and profitable life. Individuals following the Mediterranean eating regimen have been connected to a lower danger of Alzheimer's malady and malignancy, better generally speaking cardiovascular wellbeing, and an all-inclusive life expectancy. A Mediterranean style eating regimen is joined by a way of life. The way of life has many things that complete the eating routine. It incorporates a lot of exercise, not smoking, drinking in moderation, and having an enthusiasm for your family and life. This is a genuinely effective methodology for keeping up a solid life. The basic premise of this eating routine is that you eat a considerable measure of vegetables, fruits, cereals, nuts, and whole grains. You eat fish or meat scarcely. The omission of meat lessens your hazard of malignancy. You eat some bread. These are a few of the fundamental things that this eating regimen is all about.

The other portion of the Mediterranean eating regimen is the social component. You eat with your loved ones, family, and companions. You profit by the nourishment that you get and you savor your life. You eat inwardly back and center. Your family and companions appreciate it and they likewise figure out how to appreciate it. You meet a few people who are like-minded and you progress toward becoming a family. You get to appreciate your life since you're living it to the most astounding extent conceivable.

You can't take in the Mediterranean eating routine truly unless you be mindful of the exercise, the moderation, and being with the individuals who make it an occurrence to appreciate life. This is for the most part an approach of life. In the event that you need to accomplish the full advantages let this be the best way you choose to live your life. For the most part the general public who are doing it go to the gatherings that are as a rule home based. They have fun, they do things under the sun, and they do issues with their families and clan. They make a decent attempt to live in that sort of setting as opposed to the conventional social environment that a great many people are ordinarily in.

The last piece of the Mediterranean eating regimen is the way of life. One of the things that can be exceptionally harming is the way that you don't chat with your folks sufficiently. You don't get yourself the chance to hear your companions talk about the things that they appreciate, the things that they comprehend, and the things that they be in a position to do for themselves. They appreciate listening to you talk approximately the things that you appreciate, the things that you comprehend, and the things that you can do for yourself. Planning an occasion to get together so you can talk with your companions about your most loved subjects and every one of the underlying intricacies of your life is an essential piece on the way to accomplish the full advantages of the Mediterranean eating routine.

Crunchy Chickpeas

Preparation Time: 5 minutes

Cooking Time: 10 minutes

Servings: 2

Ingredients:

- ¼ cup chickpeas, canned
- 1 tablespoon avocado oil
- 1 teaspoon ground paprika

Directions:

1. Line the baking tray with baking paper.
2. Mix up chickpeas with ground paprika and avocado oil and transfer the mixture in the tray. Flatten it gently.
3. Bake the chickpeas for 10 minutes at 400F. Stir them every 2 minutes.

Nutrition: 103 calories, 5.1g protein, 16.1g carbohydrates, 2.5g fat, 5.1g fiber, 0mg cholesterol, 7mg sodium, 265mg potassium.

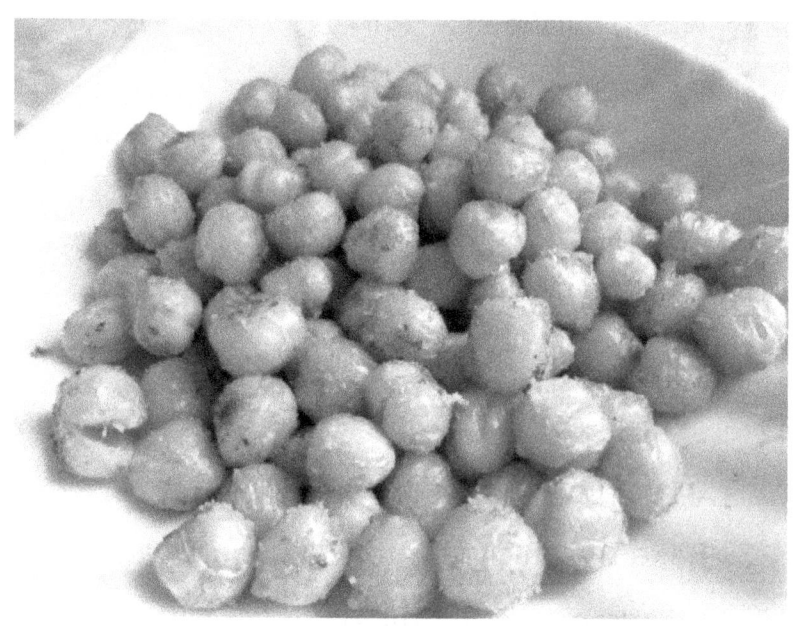

Stuffed Dates

Preparation Time: 5 minutes

Cooking Time: 0 minutes

Servings: 4

Ingredients:

- 4 dates, pitted
- 4 walnuts

Directions:

1. Fill the dates with walnuts.

Nutrition: 75 calories, 1.5g protein, 7g carbohydrates, 5g fat, 1.4g fiber, 0mg cholesterol, 0mg sodium, 54mg potassium.

Almond Gazpacho

Preparation Time: 15 minutes

Cooking Time: 0 minutes

Servings: 4

Ingredients:

- ½ cup almonds
- 1 cup cucumbers, chopped
- ½ teaspoon minced garlic
- 3 oz. water, warm
- 2 oz. chives, chopped
- 1 tablespoon sunflower oil
- ¼ cup fresh dill, chopped
- ¼ cup plain yogurt

Directions:

1. Put all ingredients in the blender and blend until smooth.
2. Cool the cooked gazpacho in the fridge for 10-15 minutes.

Nutrition: 127 calories, 4.6g protein, 7g carbohydrates, 9.9g fat, 2.4g fiber, 1mg cholesterol, 19mg sodium, 304mg potassium.

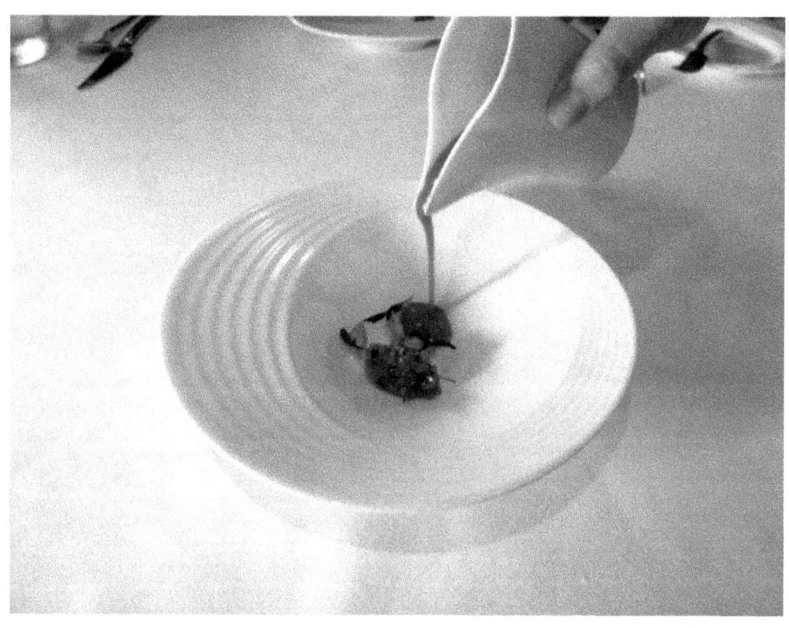

Turkey Chowder

Preparation Time: 5 minutes

Cooking Time: 20 minutes

Servings: 2

Ingredients:

- ½ cup ground turkey
- ¼ cup leek, chopped
- 1 teaspoon dried rosemary
- 1 cup of water
- 1 cup plain yogurt
- 1 teaspoon olive oil

Directions:

1. Roast the ground turkey with olive oil in the pan for 10 minutes. Stir well.
2. Then add all remaining ingredients and close the lid.
3. Cook the chowder for 10 minutes more on the medium heat.

Nutrition: 277 calories, 29.8g protein, 10.6g carbohydrates, 13g fat, 0.5g fiber, 92mg cholesterol, 180mg sodium, 536mg potassium.

PASTA AND COUSCOUS

Spaghetti Carbonara

Preparation time: 10 minutes

Cooking time: 25 minutes

Servings: 2

Ingredients

- Spaghetti 160 g
- Pancetta 120 g
- Hard cheese 50 g
- Egg yolk 2 pieces
- Salt to taste
- Freshly ground black pepper to taste

Directions:

1. Bring well-salted water to a boil. Cook spaghetti to al dente. Save a little broth from the paste; you may need it. Drain the rest.
2. While preparing the pasta, heat the pan and fry the pancetta on it until golden, remove from heat.

3. In a small bowl, beat the yolks with grated cheese until smooth.
4. Return the pan with the pancetta to a small fire, add about 50 ml of the broth from the pasta, throw the spaghetti there and mix well until the boiling stops. Most of the water should boil.
5. Remove the pan from the heat and add the yolks with cheese and mix quickly until the yolks thicken. If the sauce seems too thick, add a little more paste broth. Pepper and salt to taste, serve.

Nutrition: Calories: 702 Protein: 18 g Fat: 14 g Carbs: 33 g

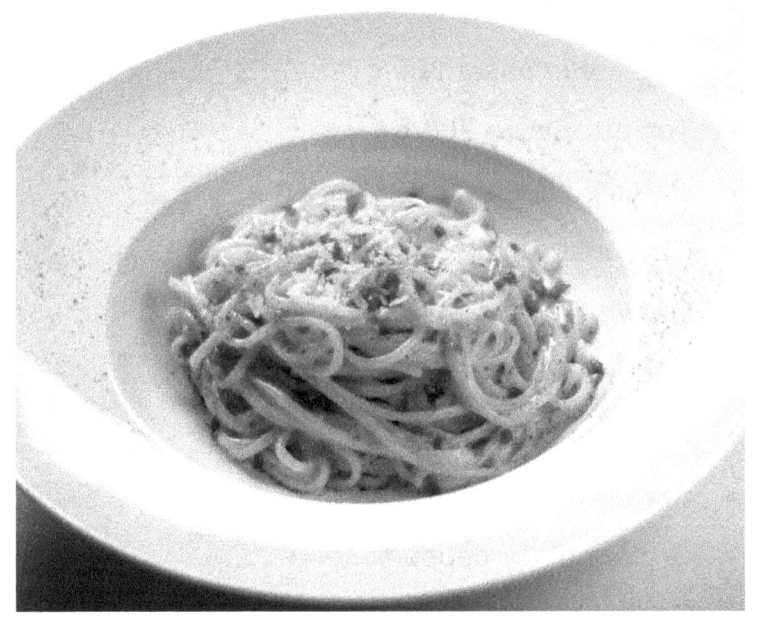

Tagliatelle Pasta

Preparation time: 15 minutes

Cooking time: 30 minutes

Servings: 4

Ingredients

- Chanterelles 200 g
- Tagliatelle pasta 200 g
- Tomato Sauce 200 g
- Garlic 2 cloves
- Olive oil 20 ml
- Dry white wine 30 ml
- Butter 10 g
- Parmesan Cheese 50 g
- Saltto taste
- Ground black pepperto taste

Directions:

1. Heat olive oil in a pan with a thick bottom, add a couple of whole cloves of garlic, add chanterelles (pre-washed and well-dried).
2. Fry the chanterelles 5-7 minutes until golden brown, pour in white wine, evaporate.

3. Then pour the tomato sauce and simmer for about 5 minutes. At the end, add butter, salt and pepper.
4. Add the paste cooked al-dente to the sauce and mix. Serve garnished with sliced parmesan and parsley.

Nutrition: Calories: 360 Protein: 18 Grams Fat: 16Grams Carbs: 32 Grams

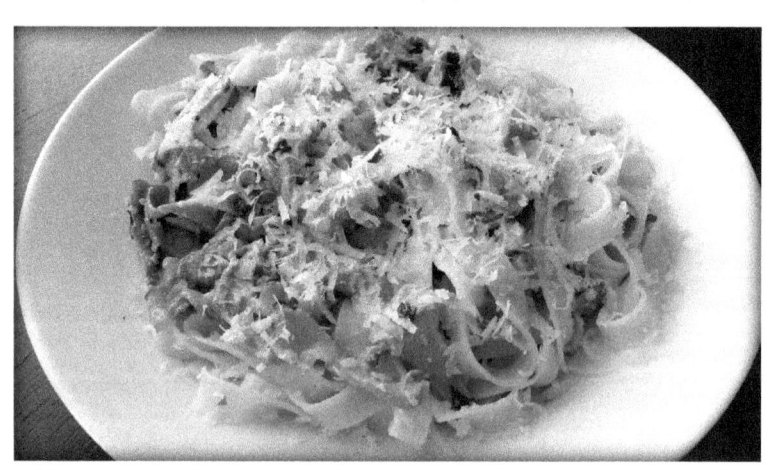

Pasta "Verochka"

Preparation time: 5 minutes

Cooking time: 20 minutes

Servings: 2

Ingredients

- Spaghetti 300 g
- Cream 33% 200 ml
- Lightly salted trout 100 g
- Grated Parmesan Cheese 50 g
- Dried oregano to taste
- Dried basil to taste

Directions:

1. Boil spaghetti - or other suitable pasta - until cooked, following the time indicated on the package. You do not need to salt water - the salt will give the fish.
2. Meanwhile, finely chop the red fish - not necessarily trout, any. And its quantity may be different - if only the fish had no more pasta.
3. Heat the cream in a pan (it is better to take fatter) and add fish to them. Keep on fire, stirring

constantly and, most importantly, not boiling. When the fish loses color, you can remove the pan from the heat.

4. Throw the prepared pasta into a colander and add to the sauce. Or add the sauce to the paste - as anyone is more familiar and convenient. Add oregano and basil, mix.
5. Sprinkle the paste spread on the plates with grated Parmesan.

Nutrition: Calories: 687 Protein: 18 Grams Fat: 14 Grams Carbs: 33 Grams

Pasta e Patate

Preparation time: 15 minutes

Cooking time: 30 minutes

Servings: 3

Ingredients

- Bacon 140 g
- Onions 80 g
- Spaghetti 240 g
- Potato400 g
- Parmesan Cheese 80 g
- Olive oil 30 ml
- Freshly ground black pepper to taste
- Salt to taste

Directions:

1. Fry the bacon in a dry skillet. Add olive oil and fry finely chopped onions, not until golden brown.
2. Add chopped potatoes to the onion, fry and add water to the onion. Cook until al dente, 5-10 minutes.
3. Break the spaghetti, toss it to the potatoes, add water, continue cooking until the spaghetti is

ready. Pour a little water over the entire cooking process so that a little liquid is left in the finale, sufficient to make a sauce.
4. In the finale add grated parmesan, olive oil, freshly ground black pepper, mix well

Nutrition: Calories: 615 Protein: 18 Grams Fat: 29 Grams Carbs: 33 Grams

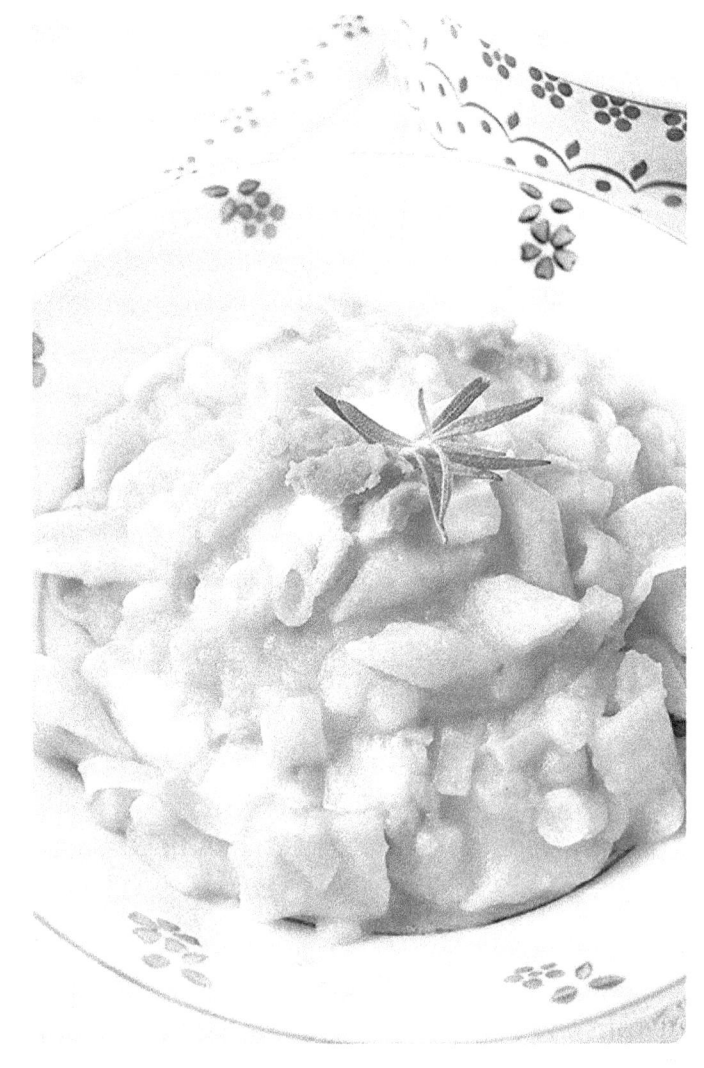

Pasta with Fresh Tomatoes

Preparation time: 15 minutes

Cooking time: 30 minutes

Servings: 3

Ingredients

- Tagliatelle pasta 200 g
- Tomatoes 1 piece
- 5 black olives
- Garlic 2 cloves
- Olive oil 50 ml

Directions:

1. Boil the paste in salted boiling water.
2. Simultaneously in 1 tablespoon of olive oil, lightly fry the garlic and sliced olives.
3. Dice the fresh tomatoes and add to the garlic and olives. Cooking tomatoes is not necessary, they should only warm up.
4. Slightly salt and pepper the sauce.
5. Drain the water and combine the pasta with the sauce.
6. Put the pasta in a plate and lightly pour olive oil.

Nutrition: Calories: 667 Protein: 18 Grams Fat: 52 Grams Carbs: 33 Grams

Spaghetti Carbonara With Chicken

Preparation time: 5 minutes

Cooking time: 30 minutes

Servings: 2

Ingredients

- Durum wheat spaghetti 300 g
- Cream 100 ml
- Garlic 2 cloves
- Chicken egg 3 pieces
- Basil to taste
- Sesame seeds 15 g
- Salt to taste
- Olive oil 3 tablespoons
- Parmesan Cheese 50 g
- Chicken fillet 200 g

Directions:

1. Finely chop the chicken fillet and fry in olive oil until tender.
2. Peel the garlic, chop finely and add to the chicken. Fry it all together for 1-2 minutes. Then add

cream, salt to taste. Stew on low heat so that the cream does not curl.
3. Add a spoonful of olive oil to boiling water, salt to taste to taste. Cooking spaghetti to al dente.
4. Cooking the sauce. To do this, beat the eggs, then add basil, salt, sesame and grated parmesan.
5. Once the spaghetti is ready, we discard them in a colander, then - in a pan with chicken and garlic, pour everything in the resulting sauce and simmer for another 2-3 minutes over low heat.

Nutrition: Calories: 624 Protein: 18 Grams Fat: 28 Grams Carbs: 33 Grams

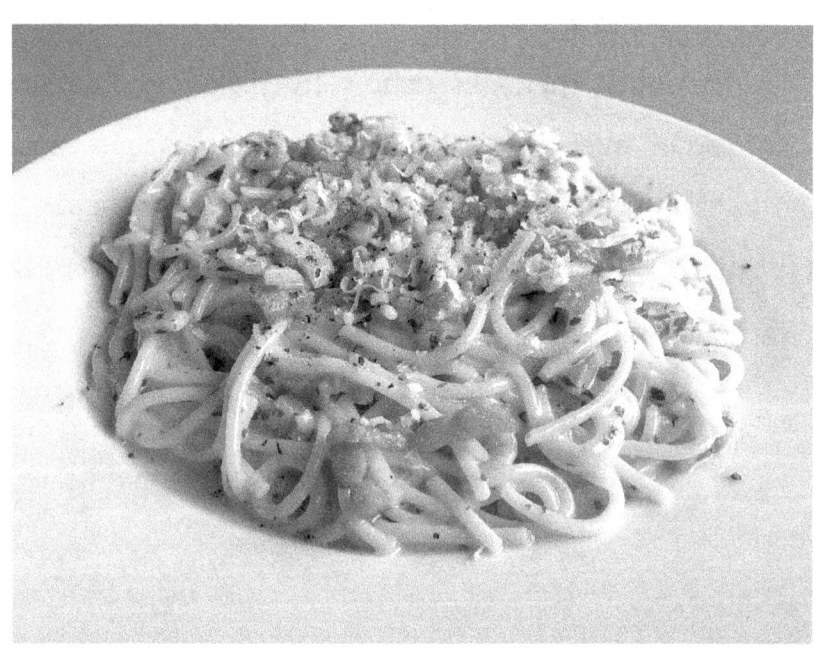

Carbonara With Fettuccine

Preparation time: 10 minutes

Cooking time: 25 minutes

Servings: 4

Ingredients

- Fettuccine Pasta 500 g
- Bacon 8 slices
- 4 eggs
- Grated Parmesan Cheese 50 g
- Cream 315 ml

Directions:

1. Cut the bacon into thin strips and fry in a pan over medium heat until crisp. Lay on a paper towel.
2. Put the pasta in a pot of boiling salted water and cook until cooked. Drain and return to pan.
3. While the pasta is boiling, beat the eggs with cream and parmesan until smooth. Add the bacon and mix well. Pour the sauce into a hot paste and mix well.

4. Return to a frying pan to a very small fire and simmer a little less than 1 minute until the sauce thickens slightly.

Nutrition: Calories: 916 Protein: 18 Grams Fat: 41 Grams Carbs: 33 Grams

Fast Spaghetti Carbonara

Preparation time: 5 minutes

Cooking time: 30 minutes

Servings: 3

Ingredients

- Spaghetti 80 g
- Bacon 40 g
- Cream 35% 50 ml
- Chicken egg 1 piece
- Dry white wine 20 ml
- Grana padano cheese 23 g

Directions:

1. We put spaghetti in boiling water, cook for 12 minutes, put it in a sieve.
2. At the chicken egg, we separate the yolk from the protein, mix the yolks with animal cream, grana padano cheese, and pepper.
3. Cut the bacon with a large plate into large plates, fry in butter, add dry white wine and olive oil.

4. Into the fried bacon with wine and oil we introduce ready-made spaghetti, add the mass with egg and cream, mix quickly

Nutrition: Calories: 847 Protein: 18 Grams Fat: 49 Grams Carbs: 33 Grams

Pasta with Greens

Preparation Time: 35 Minutes
Servings: 8
Ingredients

- Swiss chard – 1 bunch (remove the stems)
- Oil packed sun-dried tomatoes – ½ cup (chopped)
- Green olives – ½ cup (chopped and pitted)
- Fresh parmesan cheese – ¼ cup (grated)
- Dry fusilli pasta – 1 (16 ounce) package
- Olive oil – 2 tablespoons
- Kalamata olives – ½ cup (chopped and pitted)
- Garlic – 1 clove (minced)

Directions:

1. Cook pasta in lightly salted water for 10 to 12 minutes until al dente then drain.
2. Put the chard in a microwave safe bowl, fill with water until it is about ½ filled with water. Cook on high in the microwave for about 5 minutes until the chard is limp then drain.
3. Over medium heat, heat the oil in a skillet. Stir in the oil, the sun-dried tomatoes, green olives, kalamata olives and garlic.

4. Mix in the chard the cook and stir until the mixture is tender.
5. Toss with the pasta and sprinkle with parmesan cheese to serve.

Nutrition: Calories: 296; Fat: 9.7 g; Cholesterol: 2 mg; Sodium: 467 mg; Carbohydrates: 44.6 g; Protein: 9.6 g; Calcium: 66 mg; Iron: 3 mg; Potassium: 329 mg.

Tips

You can substitute the pasta with another any other that you like.

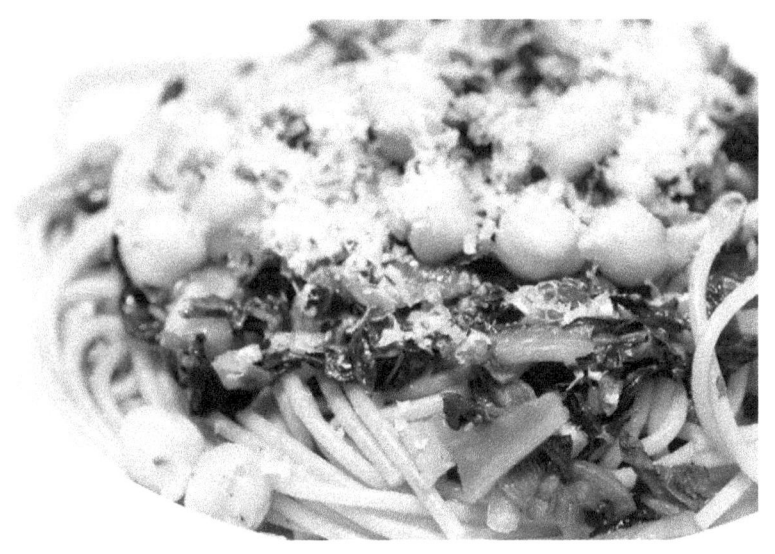

Harvest Pasta

Preparation time: 35 minutes

Cooking time: 4 minutes

Servings: 6

Ingredients

- Kalamata olives – 1/3 cup (pitted)
- Garlic – 2 cloves (minced)
- White sugar – 1 tablespoon or more to taste
- Dried oregano – 1 teaspoon
- Vegetarian burger crumbs – ¾ cup
- Diced tomatoes – 2 (14.5 ounce) cans
- Bottled roasted red peppers – 1/3 cup (chopped)
- Balsamic vinegar – 1 ½ tablespoons
- Olive oil – 2 tablespoons
- Black pepper to taste
- Penne pasta – 1 pound

Directions:

1. In a large saucepan, stir the olives, garlic, sugar, oregano, tomatoes, red pepper, vinegar. Bring this to simmer for about 20 to 30 minutes over medium high-heat before reducing to medium-

low and let simmer until the sauce starts to thicken.

2. In a large pot, pour lightly salted water and boil over high heat. Once the water is boiling, put in the penne pasta and leave to boil.
3. Cook the pasta uncovered for about 11 minutes and remember to stir occasionally until the pasta is al-dente. After this drain.
4. Once the tomato sauce is done, pour it into the blender no more than halfway full. Hold down the lid and carefully start the blender using a few pulses to get the sauce moving before leaving it on to puree. Afterwards, puree until the mixture is smooth, then return to the pot.
5. Stir in the burger crumbles and simmer until it is hot. Then pour the finished sauce over the penne pasta to serve.

Nutrition: Calories: 392; Fat: 8.8 g; Cholesterol: 0 mg; Carbohydrates: 64.9 g; Protein: 13.4 g; Iron: 6 mg; Calcium: 72 mg; Potassium: 345 mg.

Tips

You can also use a stick blender to puree the sauce in the pot until it is smooth.

Pollo Mediterranean

Preparation time: 25 minutes

Cooking time: 10 minutes

Servings: 4

Ingredients

- Olive oil – 2 tablespoons
- Garlic – 3 cloves (minced)
- Ground black pepper – ½ teaspoon
- Sun-dried tomatoes packed in oi – ¼ cup (chopped and drained)
- Dry white wine – ½ cup
- Chicken tenders – 12 (sliced into strips)
- Salt – ½ teaspoon
- Italian seasoning – 1 tablespoon
- Green olives – 2 tablespoons (sliced)
- Fresh parsley – 2 tablespoons (chopped)
- Sour cream – ½ cup
- Salt – ½ teaspoon
- Milk – 1 cup
- Cornstarch – 1 ½ teaspoons
- Water – ¼ cup

Directions:

1. In a skillet and over medium heat, heat olive oil. Place chicken and garlic in the pan. Season with pepper, Italian seasoning and ½ teaspoon of salt.
2. Stir in the olives, wine, parsley, tomatoes and olives then reduce heat to a low and continue cooking until the chicken is no longer pink at the center. Remove and place chicken on a late with the sauce still in the pan. Stir into the remaining sauce ½ teaspoon of sauce.
3. In a small bowl, whisk cornstarch and water together. Increase heat to the medium and whisk in the cornstarch mixture. Continue stirring until the sauce has thickened. Serve the sauce with chicken.

Nutrition: Calories: 392; Fat: 19.7 g; Cholesterol: 111 mg; Carbohydrates: 9.2 g; Protein: 38 g; Calcium: 157 mg; Potassium: 590 mg.

Tips

You can use artichoke in the cooking.

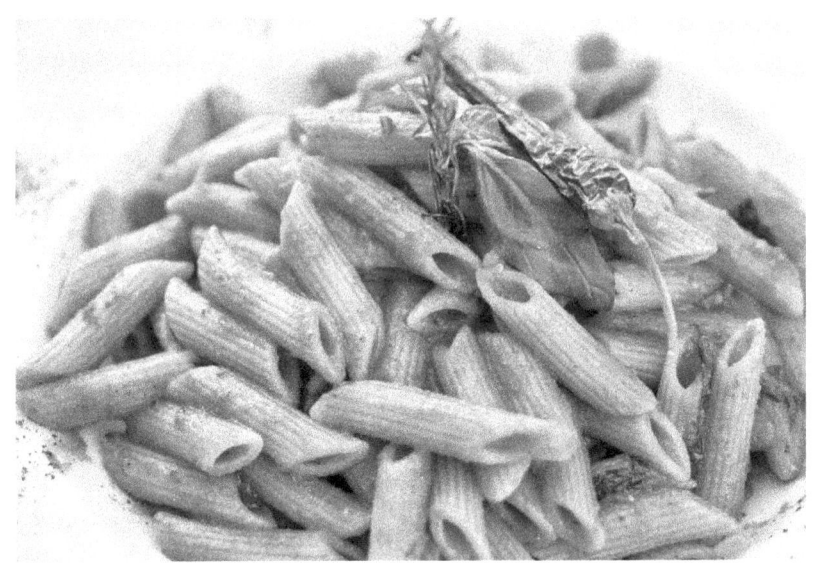

Pasta Fagioli Soup

Preparation time: 25 minutes

Cooking time: 35 minutes

Servings: 6

Ingredients:

- Water – 3 cups
- Crisp cooked bacon – 8 slices (crumbled)
- Dried parsley- 1 tablespoon
- Garlic – 1 tablespoon (minced)
- Garlic powder – 1 teaspoon
- Ground black pepper – ½ teaspoon
- Salt- 1 ½ teaspoon
- Dried basil – ½ teaspoon
- Tomato sauce – 1 (8 ounce) can
- Seashell pasta – ½ pound
- Great Northern beans – 2 (14 ounce) cans (undrained)
- Chicken broth – 2 (14.5 ounce) can
- Diced tomatoes – 1 (29 ounce) can
- Chopped spinach – 1(14 ounce) can (drained)

Directions:

1. Combine all the other ingredients apart from pasta in a large stock pot to cook and boil. Let simmer for about 40 minutes.
2. Add pasta and cook with the pot uncovered until the pasta is tender. This should take approximately 10 minutes.
3. Serve.

Nutrition: Calories: 288; Fat: 3.6 g; Cholesterol: 7 mg; carbohydrates: 48.5 g; Protein: 15.8 mg; Iron: 5 mg; Calcium: 100 mg; Potassium: 701 mg

Tip

You can substitute half of the canned ingredients for better nutritional outcomes.

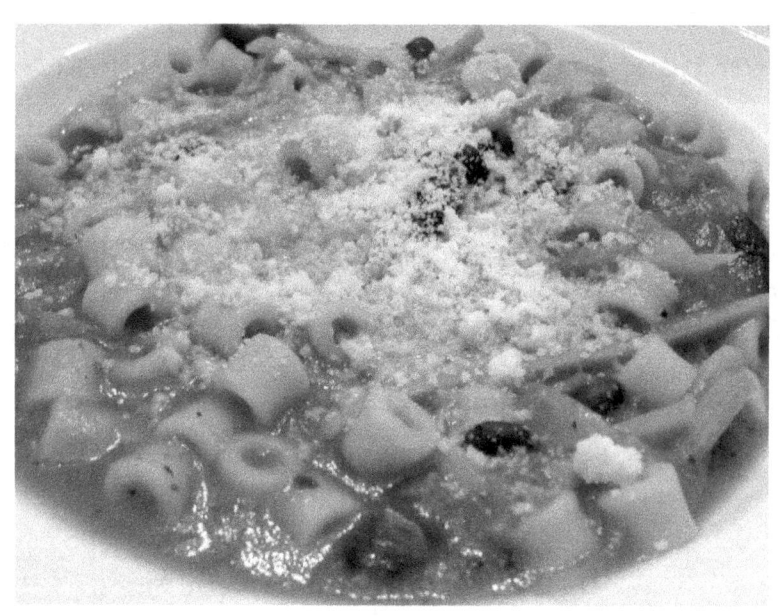

Pasta al Mediterraneo

Preparation time: 25 minutes

Cooking time: 15 minutes

Servings: 6

Ingredients

- Perciatelli pasta – 1 pound
- Pine nuts – 3 tablespoons (lightly roasted)
- Fresh parsley – 2 tablespoons (chopped)
- Lemon – 1 (juiced)
- Can tuna – 2 (5 ounce) package (drained)
- Kalamata olives – 12 (pitted and sliced)
- Garlic – 1 clove (crushed)
- Fresh basil – 4 ounces (chopped)
- Olive oil – 6 tablespoons
- Feta cheese – 2 ounces (optional)

Directions:

1. Cook pasta in a large bowl of slightly salted water until al dente. Meanwhile, mix in a large bowl, olives, garlic, basil, tuna, pine nuts, parsley and crumbled feta cheese.

2. Drain the pasta. If the plan is to serve cold, then rinse the pasta with cold water until it is no longer hot. In a large bowl, place pasta together with lemon juice and olive oil. Stir into the pasta mixture, the tuna mixture.
3. Serve hot or cold.

Nutrition: Calories: 519; Fat: 22 g; Cholesterol: 21 mg; Sodium: 255 mg; Carbohydrates: 59.5 g; Protein: 24.2 g; Calcium: 122 mg; Potassium: 370 mg.

Tips.

If possible, use fresh lemon juice instead of bottled ones.

Tomato Basil Penne Pasta

Preparation time: 45 minutes

Cooking time: 20 minutes

Servings: 4

Ingredients

- Basil oil – 1 tablespoon
- Garlic – 3 cloves (minced)
- Pepper jack cheese – 1 cup
- Parmesan cheese – ¼ cup (grated)
- Basil oil – 1 tablespoon
- Grape tomatoes – 1 pint (halved)
- Mozzarella cheese – 1cup (shredded)
- Fresh basil – 1 tablespoon (minced)

Directions:

1. Over high heat, bring a large pot of water to boil. Cook pasta in the boiling water for about 11 minutes until al dente, then drain.
2. In a large skillet and over medium-high heat, heat the basil and olive oil. Cook garlic in oil until soft. Afterwards, add tomatoes, reduce the heat to a medium and leave to dimmer for 10 minutes.

3. Stir in the mozzarella, parmesan cheese and pepper jack. When the cheese begins to melt, mix in the cooked penne pasta. Season with fresh basil.

Nutrition: Calories: 502; Fat: 24.8 g; Cholesterol: 58 mg; Sodium: 462 mg; Carbohydrates: 47.1 g; Protein: 24.1 g; Calcium: 474 mg; Potassium: 311 mg.

Tip

If basil oil is unavailable, use 2 tablespoons of olive oil.

Whole Wheat Pasta Toss

Preparation time: 25 minutes

Cooking time: 30 minutes

Servings: 8

Ingredients

- Olive oil – 1/3 cup
- Marinated artichoke hearts – 1 (8 ounce) jar (drained)
- Kalamata olives – ¼ cup (pitted and quartered)
- Feta cheese – ½ cup (crumbled)
- Whole wheat penne pasta – 1 (1 pound) package
- Garlic – 4 large cloves (pressed)
- Pickled red peppers – 7 (cut into strips)
- Fresh spinach leaves – 2 cups

Directions:

1. Fill a large bowl with lightly salted water and bring to boil. Put in the penne and continue to boil. Cook the pasta uncovered, stirring occasionally for 8 minutes or until al dente, then drain.
2. In a large non-stick skillet and over medium heat, heat olive oil, the cook and stir in garlic into the

hot oil for about 30 seconds until it is fragrant, for about 5 minutes. Gently fold the spinach into the mixture and stir just until slightly wilted and dark green.

3. Remove the mixture from heat and stir in the penne pasta until it is thoroughly combined; lightly toss pasta mixture in with the feta steam, cover the skillet with a lid and let the vegetables and pasta steam for about 10 minutes before serving.

Nutrition: Calories: 367; Fat :14.7 g; Cholesterol: 8 mg; Sodium: 347 mg; Carbohydrates: 47.4 g; Protein: 12.9 g; Iron: 1 mg; Calcium: 60 mg; Potassium: 58 mg.

Quick Mediterranean Pasta

Preparation time: 25 minutes

Cooking time: 10 minutes

Servings: 6

Ingredients

- Breadcrumbs – ¼ cup
- Dried basil – 1 teaspoon
- Spaghetti – 8 ounces
- Dried oregano – 1 teaspoon
- Olive oil – 1 tablespoon

Directions:

1. Boil slightly salted water in a large pot, put spaghetti in it and cook until al dente. Rinse and cool with water, then drain well.
2. Mix the breadcrumbs, basil, oregano and cooked pasta in a large bowl. Pour as much olive oil as you would like over the mixture and serve.

Nutrition: Calories: 178; Fat: 3.1 g; Cholesterol: 0 mg; Sodium: 35 mg; Carbohydrate: 31.4 g; Protein: 5.5 g; Iron: 2 mg; Calcium: 25 mg; Potassium: 104 mg.

Tips

You can always experiment with the recipe

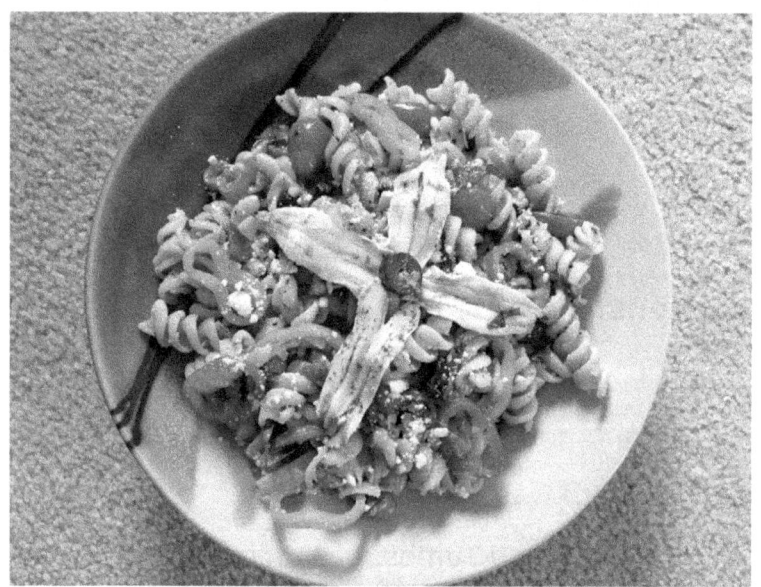

Mediterranean Fish and Pasta Stew

Preparation time: 20 minutes

Cooking time: 30 minutes

Servings: 4

Ingredients

- Onions – 2 (chopped)
- Crushed tomatoes – 1 (28 ounce) can
- Fresh parsley – ½ cup (chopped)
- Worcestershire sauce – 2 tablespoons
- Paprika – 1 teaspoon
- Dry pasta – 3 ounces
- Garlic – 4 cloves (minced)
- Olive oil – 1 tablespoon
- Water – 6 cups
- Fresh cilantro – ½ cup (chopped)
- Ground cinnamon – 1 teaspoon
- Cod fillets – 1 ½ pounds (cubed)
- Salt to taste
- Ground black pepper – 1 tablespoon

Directions:

1. In a large pot, sauté the onions and garlic in the olive oil for 5 minutes over medium heat while stirring constantly.
2. Add tomatoes with the liquid, parsley, water and cilantro. Bring the mixture to boil and reduce heat to low and simmer for about 15 minutes.
3. Stir in the Worcestershire sauce, paprika, cinnamon and fish, the simmer over medium heat for 10 minutes. Add the pasta and simmer for about 8 minutes more or until the pasta is tender.
4. Season with salt and ground pepper to taste.

Nutrition: Calories: 237; Fat: 4.2 g; Cholesterol: 66 mg; Sodium: 300 mg; Carbohydrates: 26.2 g; Protein: 25.3 g; Iron: 4 mg; Calcium: 103 mg; Potassium: 1030 mg.

Tips

You can substitute some ingredients and add in some more in accordance with your taste.

Parsley Pesto Paste

Preparation time: 5 minutes

Cooking time: 15 minutes

Servings: 4

Ingredients

- 2 cups of parsley leaves
- 1/2 cup of grated parmesan cheese
- Two cloves of garlic
- 1/2 cup lemon juice
- 1/4 cup olive oil
- 1/3 cup pine nut
- Table salt to taste

Directions:

1. Put all ingredients except the parmesan cheese in a food processor then pulse until smooth.
2. Remove from the blender, add grated parmesan and gently stir.
3. Serve.

Nutrition: Calories 266, Fat 25g, Carbohydrates 6g, Protein 8g

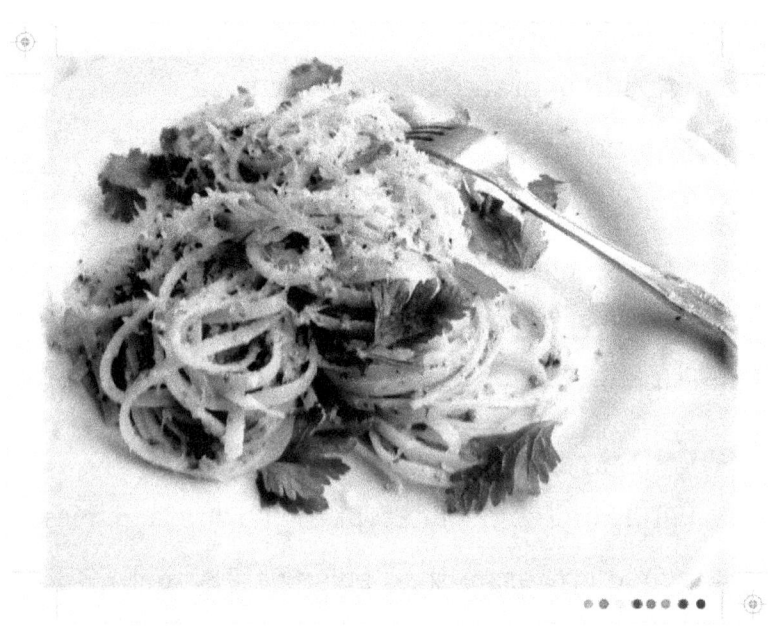

Potato in Tomato Paste

Preparation time: 25 minutes

Cooking time: 30 minutes

Servings: 4

Ingredients

- Four large cubed potatoes
- 1 Tbsp aromatic dry spices mix
- One onion, chopped
- 4 Tbsp Olive oil
- Black pepper
- One minced garlic clove
- 1 cup tomato paste
- 1 cup of water
- Chopped parsley,
- Salt

Directions:

1. Heat the olive oil in a pan over medium heat and sauté the onion until translucent.
2. Add the potatoes, the spice mixture and continue to sauté.

3. Add the garlic, tomato paste, diced tomato, water, salt and pepper, and stir.
4. Cover the pot and cook for half an hour over low heat.
5. Serve with fresh coriander.

Nutrition: Calories 312, Fat 14g, Carbohydrates 43g, Protein 6g

Hummus

Preparation time: 15 minutes

Cooking time: 10 minutes

Servings: 4

Ingredients

- 1/2 cup tahini
- 1 tsp salt
- Two cloves garlic halved
- 1 tbsp olive oil
- 2 cup canned garbanzo beans, drained
- 1/2 cup lemon juice
- 1 tbsp paprika
- 1 tsp parsley

Directions:

1. Pulse the garlic, lemon juice, garbanzos, salt, and tahini in a food processor until smooth.
2. Add this to a bowl with olive oil, paprika, and parsley.
3. Enjoy.

Nutrition: Calories 77 Fat 4.3 g Carbohydrates 8.1g Protein 2.6 g

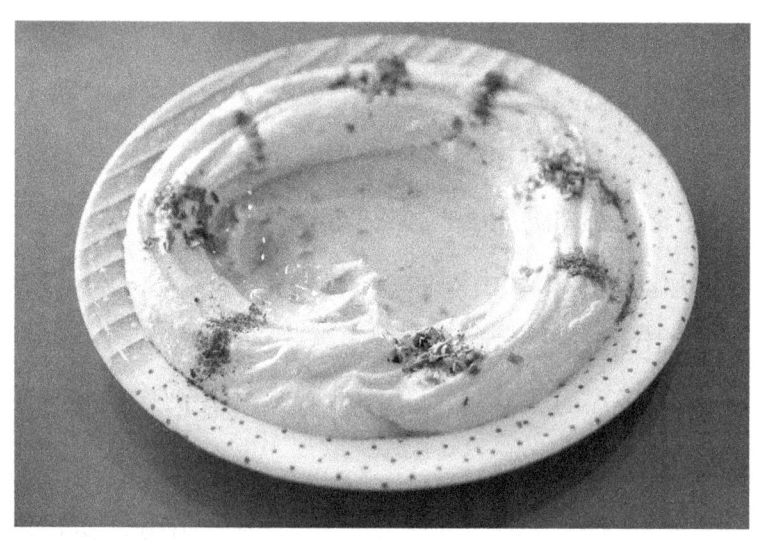

Hollandaise Sauce

Preparation time: 10 minutes

Cooking time: 5 minutes

Servings: 1

Ingredients

- One lemon (Zested and juiced)
- One tsp garlic powder
- 1/2 tsp cayenne pepper
- 1/2 cup cashew butter
- Two tsp Dijon mustard
- 1/2 cup of warm water
- 1/2 tsp ground turmeric

Directions:

1. In a food processor, put all ingredients, and then pulse until smooth.
2. Put it in a sealed container and refrigerate it for up to three days.
3. Enjoy.

Nutrition: Calories 150 Protein 6 g Fat 12 g Carbohydrates 10 g

Creamy Tahini Dip

Preparation time: 5 minutes

Cooking time: 4 minutes

Servings: 4

Ingredients

- Half a lemon (Juiced)
- One crushed garlic clove
- Salt
- 1/2 cup tahini
- 2 cups of water
- Fresh parsley, chopped
- Black pepper

Directions:

1. Put the tahini, salt, lemon juice, garlic, and a little water in a bowl then stir until the tahini becomes white and smooth.
2. Sprinkle the parsley and black pepper and serve.
3. Enjoy.

Nutrition: Calories 93 Protein 2.6 g Fat 8.1 g Carbohydrates 4.4 g

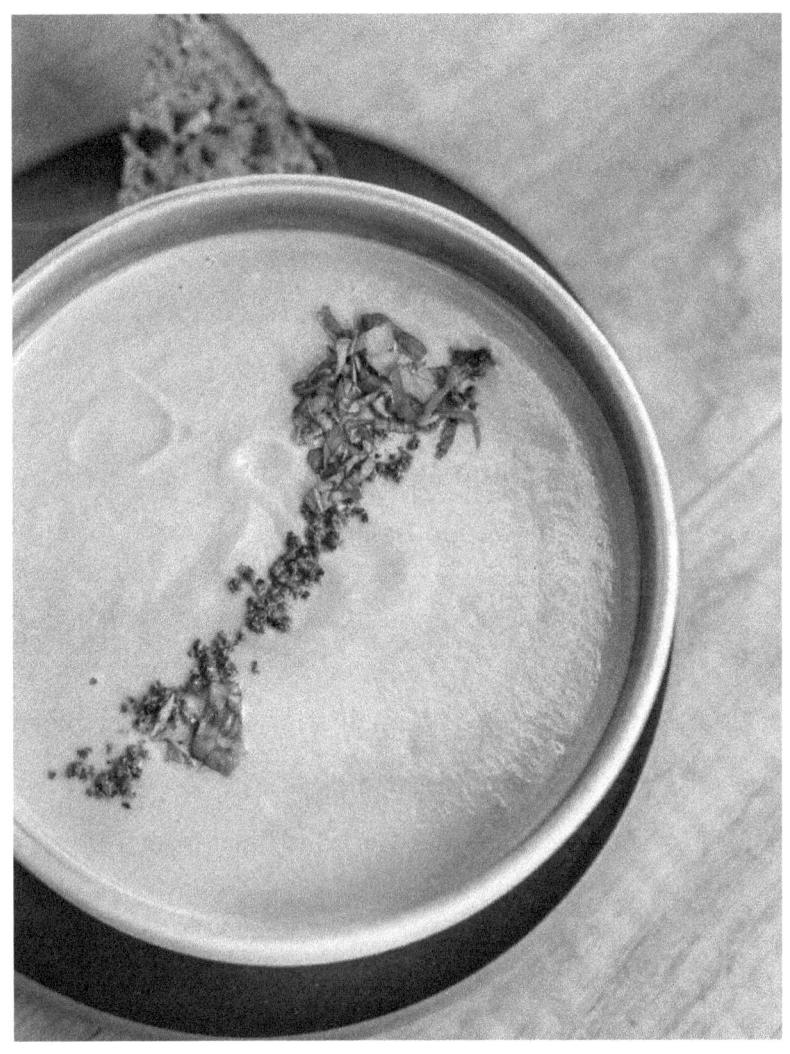

Basil Lime Dip

Preparation time: 5 minutes

Cooking time: 10 minutes

Servings: 16

Ingredients

- Ten garlic cloves, crushed
- 1/4 cup brown rice syrup
- 8 ounces hemp oil
- One tsp of sea salt
- One pinch xanthan gum
- 1 1/2 cups chopped basil,
- Six tbsp key lime juice

Directions:

1. In an airtight jar, put all the ingredients except the xanthan gum, and then shake to well.
2. Put the mixture plus the xanthan, into a blender and pulse.
3. Return the mixture in the jar.
4. Enjoy.

Nutrition: Calories 143 Cholesterol 0 mg Fat 14 g Carbohydrates 6 g

Cilantro Dip

Preparation time: 5 minutes

Cooking time: 4 minutes

Servings: 7

Ingredients:

- 12 cloves of garlic
- 4 cups cilantro leaves
- One tsp salt
- 1/2 tsp ground black pepper
- 1 cup olive oil

Directions:

1. Add all ingredients to a blender and pulse until velvety.
2. You can put in the refrigerator for up to two days.
3. Enjoy.

Nutrition: calories 230; fat 20.5 g; carbohydrates 7.1 g; protein 5 g

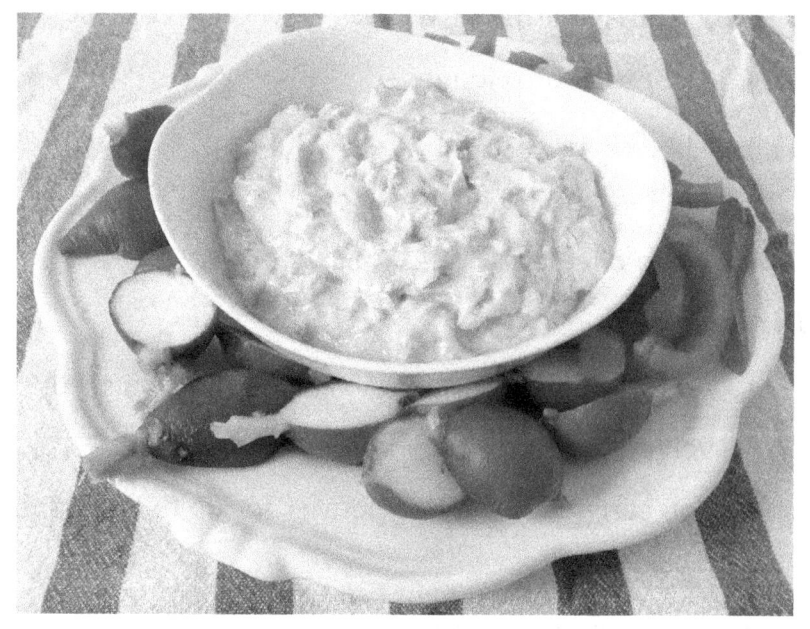

Tahini Sauce

Preparation time: 7 minutes

Cooking time: 5 minutes

Servings: 6

Ingredients:

- Four mashed garlic cloves
- Salt to taste
- 1 cup tahini paste
- 1/2 cup lemon juice
- Seven tbsp water

Directions:

1. Put all ingredients in a bowl and whisk until well combined.
2. Refrigerate up to 5 days.
3. Enjoy.

Nutrition: calories 77; fat 6.6 g; carbohydrates 3.2 g; protein 2.3 g

Arugula Salsa

Preparation time: 5 minutes

Cooking time: 20 minutes

Servings: 6

Ingredients:

- 30 Kalamata olives, pitted, quartered
- Three tbsp olive oil
- One chopped red bell pepper
- One chopped yellow bell pepper
- Two tsp fennel seeds, crushed
- 1 cup baby arugula, chopped

Directions:

1. Heat oil in a pan over medium heat.
2. Add fennel seeds and sauté until fragrant.
3. Add bell peppers and sauté until they are soft.
4. Transfer into a bowl.
5. Add salt, pepper, and arugula and stir until arugula wilts.
6. Enjoy.

Nutrition: calories 16; fat 0.1 g; carbohydrates 3.9 g; protein 0.6 g

RICE AND GRAINS

Fragrant Basmati Rice

Preparation Time: 5 minutes

Cooking Time: 17 minutes

Servings: 6

Ingredients:

- 1 cup long-grain rice
- 1 tablespoon olive oil
- 1 teaspoon dried rosemary
- 2 ½ cup water

Direction:

1. Heat the olive oil in the saucepan.
2. Add rice and roast it for 2 minutes. Stir it constantly.
3. Then add rosemary and water.
4. Stir the rice and close the lid.
5. Cook it for 15 minutes or until it soaks all water.

Nutrition: Calories: 334; Protein: 12.3g; Fat: 6.3g

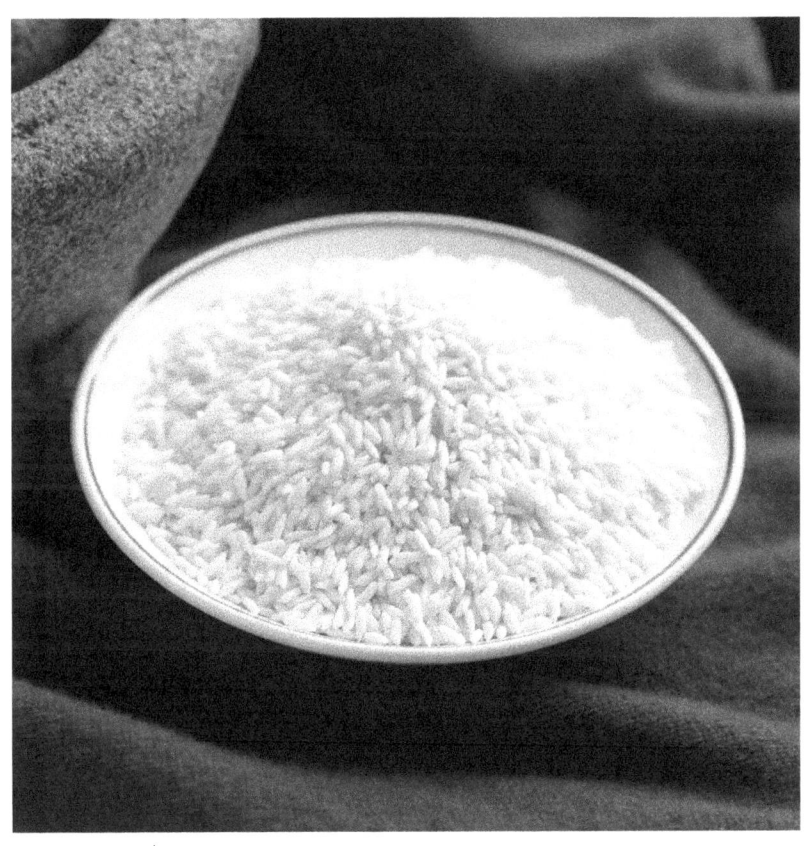

Cranberry Rice

Preparation Time: 5 minutes

Cooking Time: 20 minutes

Servings: 4

Ingredients:

- ¼ cup basmati rice
- 1 cup of organic almond milk
- 2 oz dried cranberries
- ¼ teaspoon ground cinnamon

Direction:

1. Put all ingredients in the saucepan, stir, and close the lid.
2. Cook the rice on low heat for 20 minutes.

Nutrition: Calories: 153; Protein: 12.3g; Carbs: 3.4g; Fat: 6.3g

Italian Style Wild Rice

Preparation Time: minutes

Cooking Time: 20 minutes

Servings: 6

Ingredients:

- 1 cup wild rice
- 3 cups chicken stock
- 1 teaspoon Italian seasonings
- 2 oz Feta, crumbled
- 1 tablespoon olive oil

Direction:

1. Mix wild rice with olive oil and chicken stock.
2. Close the lid and cook it for 25 minutes over the medium-low heat.
3. Then add Italian seasonings and crumbled feta.
4. Stir the rice.

Nutrition: Calories: 253; Protein: 15.3g; Carbs: 3.4g; Fat: 6.3g

Brown Rice Saute

Preparation Time: 5 minutes

Cooking Time: 20 minutes

Servings: 3

Ingredients:

- 3 oz brown rice
- 9 oz chicken stock
- 1 teaspoon curry powder
- 1 onion, diced
- 4 tablespoons olive oil

Direction:

1. Heat olive oil in the saucepan.
2. Add onion and cook it until light brown.
3. Add brown rice, curry powder, and chicken stock.
4. Close the lid and saute the rice for 15 minutes.

Nutrition: Calories: 237; Protein: 12.3g; Carbs: 3.4g; Fat: 6.3g

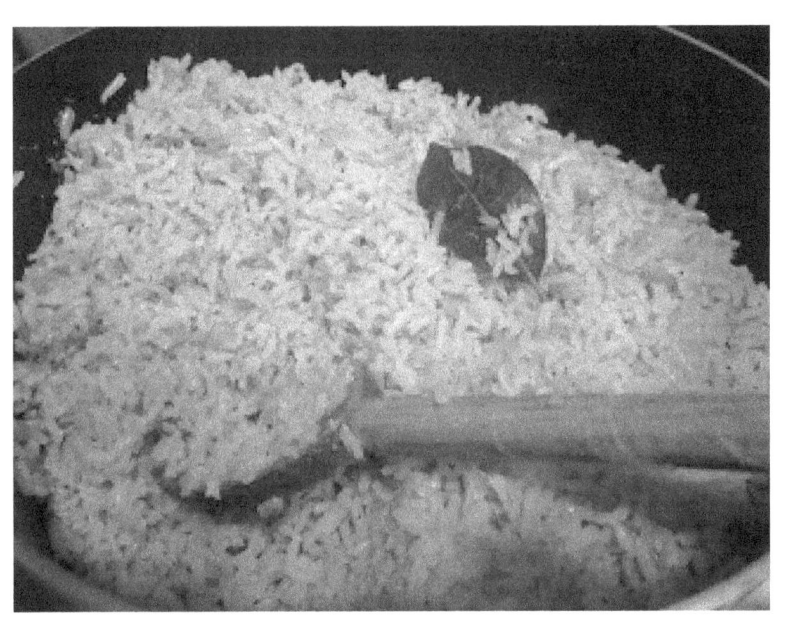

Pesto Rice

Preparation Time: 8 minutes

Cooking Time: 15 minutes

Servings: 4

Ingredients:

- ½ cup of basmati rice
    - 1.5cup of water
- 2 tablespoons pesto sauce

Direction:

1. Simmer the rice water for 15 minutes on the low heat or until the rice soaks all liquid.
2. Then mix cooked tice with pesto sauce.

Nutrition: Calories: 353; Protein: 12.3g; Carbs: 3.4g; Fat: 6.3g

Rice Salad

Preparation Time: 10 minutes

Cooking Time: 0 minutes

Servings: 4

Ingredients:

- ½ cup long-grain rice, cooked
- ½ cup corn kernels, cooked
- 1 tomato, chopped
- 1 teaspoon chili flakes
- ¼ cup plain yogurt
- 1 cucumber pickle

Direction:

1. Grate the cucumber pickle and mix it with cooked rice, corn kernels, tomato, chili flakes, and plain yogurt.

Nutrition: Calories: 153; Protein: 12.3g; Fat: 6.3g

Rice Meatballs

Preparation Time: 10 minutes

Cooking Time: 15 minutes

Servings: 20

Ingredients:

- ¼ cup Cheddar cheese, shredded
- 1 teaspoon ground black pepper
- 1 cup of basmati rice, cooked
- ¼ cup ground chicken
- 1 teaspoon olive oil

Direction:

1. In the mixing bowl, mix Cheddar cheese, ground black pepper, rice, and ground chicken.
2. Then make the balls from the mixture.
3. Heat the olive oil well and put the rice balls in the hot oil.
4. Roast the balls for 1 minute per side on high heat.
5. Then transfer the balls in the oven and bake them for 20 minutes at 360F.

Nutrition: Calories: 183; Protein: 12.3g; Fat: 6.3g

Mediterranean Paella

Preparation Time: 10 minutes

Cooking Time: 30 minutes

Servings: 6

Ingredients:

- 1 cup risotto rice
- 2 oz yellow onion, diced
- ½ teaspoon ground paprika
- 1 cup tomatoes, chopped
- 1 cup shrimps, peeled
- 1 teaspoon olive oil
- 3 cups of water

Direction:

1. Heat olive oil in the saucepan.
2. Add onion and cook it for 2 minutes.
3. Then stir well, add shrimps, ground paprika, tomatoes, and stir well.
4. Cook the ingredients for 5 minutes.
5. Add water and risotto rice. Stir well, close the lid, and cook the meal for 20 minutes on low heat.

Nutrition: Calories: 223; Protein: 12.3g; Fat: 6.3g

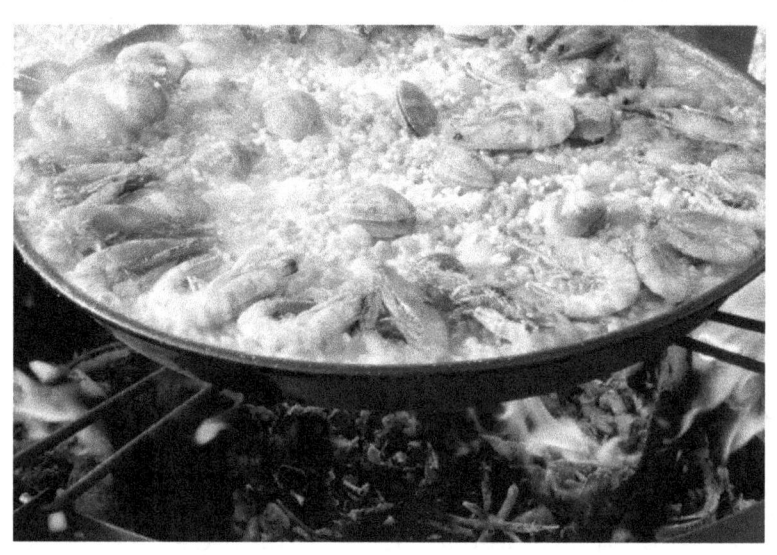

Fast Chicken Rice

Preparation Time: 10 minutes

Cooking Time: 20 minutes

Servings: 5

Ingredients:

- 1 cup basmati rice
- 3 tablespoons avocado oil
- 2.5cups chicken stock
- ½ teaspoon dried dill
- 10 oz chicken breast, skinless, boneless, chopped

Direction:

1. Mix oil with rice and roast it in the saucepan for 5 minutes over the low heat.
2. Then add chicken and chicken stock.
3. Add dill, stir the ingredients and cook the meal on medium heat for 15 minutes or until all ingredients are cooked.

Nutrition: Calories: 213; Protein: 12.3g; Fat: 6.3g

Rice Jambalaya

Preparation Time: 5 minutes

Cooking Time: 30 minutes

Servings: 8

Ingredients:

- 1 cup tomatoes, chopped
- 1 cup bell pepper, chopped
- ¼ cup carrot, chopped
- 1 teaspoon cayenne pepper
- 4 cups chicken stock
- 1 cup of basmati rice
- 2 tablespoons olive oil
- ½ cup chickpeas, cooked

Direction:

1. Melt the olive oil and add carrot, bell pepper, and tomatoes.
2. Cook the vegetables for 10 minutes on medium heat.
3. Then add chicken stock, chickpeas, and rice.
4. Add cayenne pepper and stir the meal.

5. Close the lid and cook it for 20 minutes on low heat.

Nutrition: Calories: 263; Protein: 10.3g; Carbs: 3.4g; Fat: 6.3g

Jasmine Rice with Scallions

Preparation Time: 10 minutes

Cooking Time: 10 minutes

Servings: 6

Ingredients:

- 3 tablespoons olive oil
- 1 cup jasmine rice
- 2 tablespoons scallions, chopped
- ½ teaspoon ground black pepper
- 2 teaspoons lemon juice

Direction:

1. Cook the rice according to the directions of the manufacturer.
2. Then add scallions, olive oil, ground black pepper, and lemon juice.
3. Carefully stir the meal.

Nutrition: Calories: 189; Protein: 12.3g; Fat: 6.3g

Cremini Mushrooms Pilaf

Preparation Time: 10 minutes

Cooking Time: 25 minutes

Servings: 6

Ingredients:

- 2 cups of water
- ½ cup white onion, diced
- 1 cup cremini mushrooms, chopped
- 1 cup of basmati rice
- ¼ teaspoon lime zest, grated
- 2 oz goat cheese, crumbled
- 2 tablespoons olive oil

Direction:

1. Put rice in the saucepan.
2. Add water and cook for 15 minutes over the low heat.
3. Then roast the mushrooms with olive oil, lime zest, and white onion in the skillet until they are light brown.
4. Add the cooked mushrooms in the cooked rice. Stir well.

5. Top the meal with crumbled goat cheese.

Nutrition: Calories: 193; Protein: 12.3g; Fat: 6.3g

Vegetable Rice

Preparation Time: 10 minutes

Cooking Time: 30 minutes

Servings: 6

Ingredients:

- 2 cups wild rice
- 1 teaspoon Italian seasonings
- 1 tablespoon olive oil
- ¼ cup carrot, diced
- ½ cup snap peas, frozen
- 5 cups of water

Direction:

1. Mix 4 cups of water and wild rice in the saucepan.
2. Cook the rice for 15 minutes or until the rice soaks all liquid.
3. Then heat the olive oil in the separated saucepan.
4. Add carrot and roast it until light brown.
5. Add snap peas, water, and rice.
6. Stir well and close the lid.
7. Cook the rice for 10 minutes.

Nutrition: Calories: 187; Protein: 12.3g; Fat: 4.3g

Tomato Rice

Preparation Time: 10 minutes

Cooking Time: 20 minutes

Servings: 4

Ingredients:

- 1 cup basmati rice
- 3 cups chicken stock
- 1 teaspoon ground coriander
- ¼ teaspoon dried thyme
- 2 tablespoons olive oil
- 2 tablespoons tomato paste

Direction:

1. Roast the rice with olive oil in the saucepan for 5 minutes. Stir it.
2. Then add thyme, coriander, and tomato paste.
3. Add water, mix the rice mixture, and close the lid.
4. Cook the rice for 15 minutes over the medium heat.

Nutrition: Calories: 53; Protein: 12.3g; Fat: 6.3g

Rice with Grilled Tomatoes

Preparation Time: 10 minutes

Cooking Time: 20 minutes

Servings: 6

Ingredients:

- 1 cup of basmati rice
    - cups chicken stock
- 1 teaspoon olive oil
- 2 tomatoes, roughly sliced

Direction:

1. Sprinkle the tomatoes with olive oil and grill in the preheated to 400F grill for 1 minute per side.
2. Then cook rice with chicken stock for 15 minutes.
3. Transfer the cooked rice in the bowls and top with grilled tomatoes.

Nutrition: Calories: 83; Protein: 12.3g; Fat: 6.3g

Rice and Meat Salad

Preparation Time: 10 minutes

Cooking Time: 0 minutes

Servings: 6

Ingredients:

- 1 cup white cabbage, shredded
- 1 cup long grain rice, cooked
- 8 oz beef steak, cooked, cut into the strips
- 1/3 cup plain yogurt
- 1 teaspoon salt
- 1 teaspoon chives, chopped

Direction:

1. Put cabbage and rice in the big bowl.
2. Add white rice and meat strips.
3. Then add plain yogurt, chives, and salt.
4. Stir the salad until homogenous.

Nutrition: Calories: 123; Protein: 12.3g; Fat: 6.3g

Rice Bowl

Preparation Time: 10 minutes

Cooking Time: 0 minutes

Servings: 6

Ingredients:

- 1 cup of basmati rice, cooked
- 4 oz beef sirloin, grilled
- ½ cup tomatoes, chopped
- 2 tablespoons soy sauce
- 1 teaspoon ground paprika
- 2 oz scallions, sliced

Direction:

1. Put the cooked rice in the serving bowls.
2. Add beef sirloin, tomatoes, and scallions.
3. Then sprinkle the meal with soy sauce and ground paprika.

Nutrition: Calories: 63; Protein: 12.3g; Fat: 6.3g

Zucchini Rice

Preparation Time: 10 minutes

Cooking Time: 25 minutes

Servings: 2

Ingredients:

- ½ cup of long grain rice
- cup chicken stock
- 1 zucchini, cubed
- 1 tablespoon olive oil
- 1 teaspoon curry powder
- 1 tablespoon raisins

Direction:

1. Mix rice and chicken stock in the saucepan and cook for 15 minutes or until the rice soaks the liquid.
2. Then heat the olive oil.
3. Add zucchini in the oil and roast for 5 minutes.
4. After this, sprinkle the zucchini with curry powder, add raisins and rice.
5. Carefully mix the rice and cook for 5 minutes.

Nutrition: Calories: 113; Protein: 12.3g; Fat: 4.3g

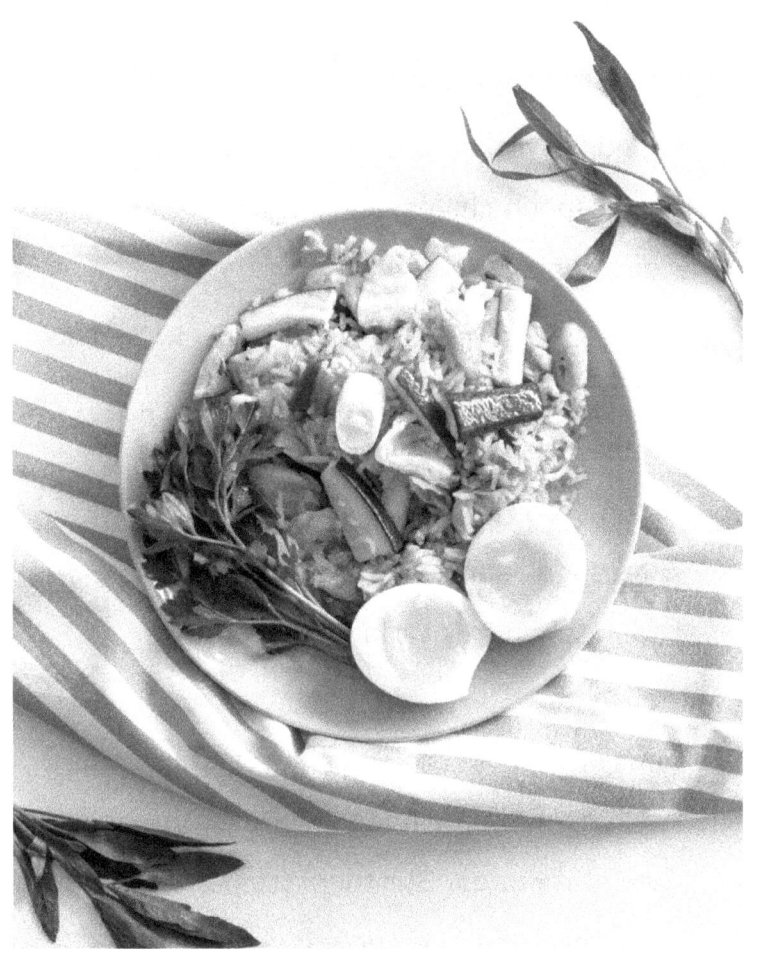

Rice Soup

Preparation time: 10 minutes

Cooking time: 20 minutes

Servings: 4

Ingredients:

- 3 cups chicken stock
- ½ pound chicken breast, shredded
- 1 tablespoon chives, chopped
- 1 egg, whisked
- ½ white onion, diced
- 1 bell pepper, chopped
- 1 tablespoon olive oil
- ¼ cup arborio rice
- ½ teaspoon salt
- 1 tablespoon fresh cilantro, chopped

Directions:

1. Pour olive oil in the stock pan and preheat it.
2. Add onion and bell pepper. Roast the vegetables for 3-4 minutes. Stir them from time to time.
3. After this, add rice and stir well.

4. Cook the ingredients for 3 minutes over the medium heat.
5. Then add chicken stock and stir the soup well.
6. Add salt and bring the soup to boil.
7. Add shredded chicken breast, cilantro, and chives. Add egg and stir it carefully.
8. Close the lid and simmer the soup for 5 minutes over the medium heat.
9. Remove the cooked soup from the heat.

Nutrition: Calories 176, Fat 6.6, Fiber 1, Protein 15.2

Rice with Prunes

Preparation Time: 5 minutes

Cooking Time: 20 minutes

Servings: 7

Ingredients:

- 1.5cup basmati rice
- 3 tablespoons organic canola oil
- 5 prunes, chopped
- ¼ cup cream cheese
- 3.5cups water
- ½ teaspoon salt

Direction:

1. Mix water and basmati rice in the saucepan and boil for 15 minutes on low heat.
2. Then add cream cheese, salt, and prunes.
3. Stir the rice carefully and bring it to boil.
4. Add organic canola oil and cook for 1 minute more.

Nutrition: Calories: 83; Protein: 12.3g; Fat: 6.3g

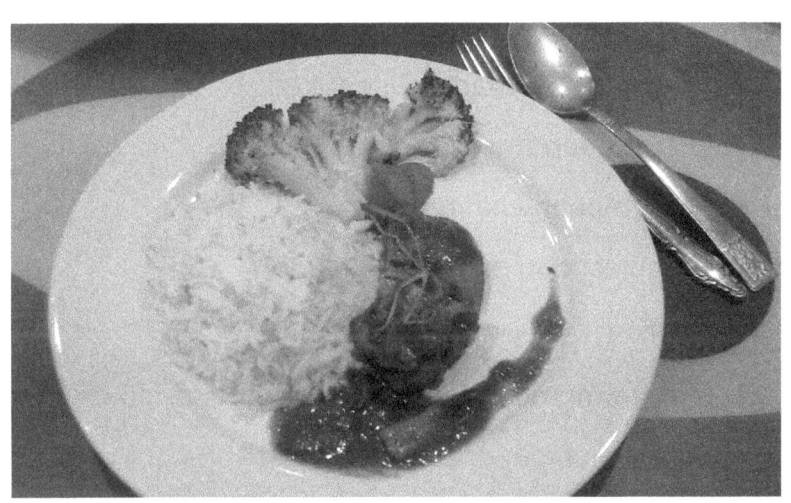

Rice and Fish Cakes

Preparation Time: 10 minutes

Cooking Time: 10 minutes

Servings: 6

Ingredients:

- 6 oz salmon, canned, shredded
- 1 egg, beaten
- ¼ cup of basmati rice, cooked
- 1 teaspoon dried cilantro
- ½ teaspoon chili flakes
- 1 tablespoon organic canola oil

Direction:

1. Mix salmon with egg, basmati rice, dried cilantro, and chili flakes.
2. Heat the organic canola oil in the skillet.
3. Make the small cakes from the salmon mixture and put in the hot oil.
4. Roast the cakes for 2 minutes per side or until they are light brown.

Nutrition: Calories: 123; Protein: 12.3g; Fat: 6.3g

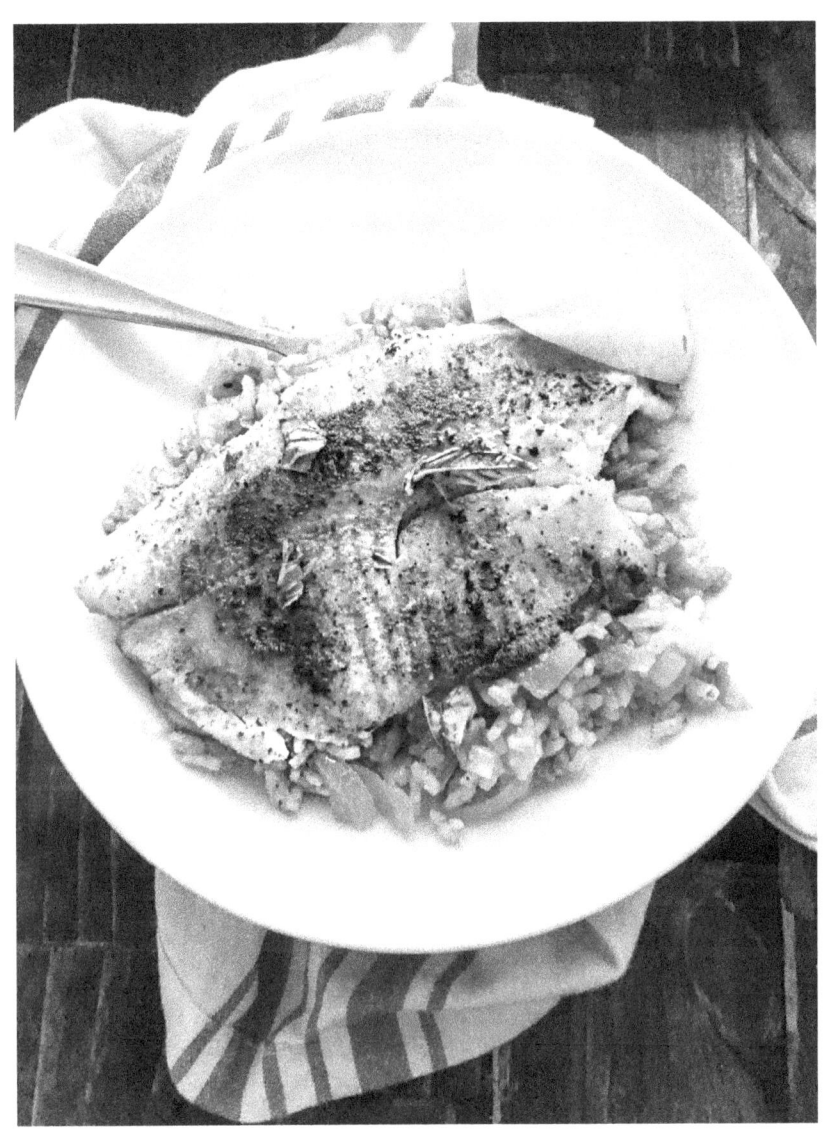

Conclusion

The Mediterranean diet considers various aspects of what "health" means. It does not just focus on what you eat but it also focuses on how you eat, who you eat with, and the activities you do in between eating. Each of these components can contribute to better health and a more fulfilling life. When we are lacking in any of these components, we tend to suffer from poor health, fatigue, depression and more. The Mediterranean diet was originally looked at because of its heart health benefits, but now it is clear to see that the traditional Mediterranean lifestyle from the 1950s was more than just a heart-healthy plan.

This book has helped you understand not only the benefits of this diet but has revealed effective tips and suggestions to help you transition into this type of diet. The changes can be made in small steps, because even the smallest change to shifting your diet to a more Mediterranean diet can have a whirlwind of benefits. You have learned how to swap the unhealthy foods you have been used to consuming with nutrient-dense and wholesome foods.

The Mediterranean diet is more than what you eat; it is a way of living. This diet reflects the true definition of what a diet should be. It encourages eating healthy nutritious foods, while also emphasizing the importance of physical activity and spending time with those we care about. The Mediterranean diet has been studied for decades and each time it seems a new benefit of this diet comes to light.

What needs to be done is adopting a new way of looking at food and mealtimes. Our world today stresses working harder and longer which means there is little time for enjoying meals. If we can change our perspective to see that the food, we eat is what makes us more efficient and productive, then we would be able to more easily change the way we eat.

This book has introduced you to what the Mediterranean diet is. It has helped you understand that this isn't your typical diet. That instead, the Mediterranean diet is about changing into a lifestyle that will bring you better health and happiness. This book has provided you with some of the findings from scientific research that supports the diet's benefits. You have learned that the diet consists of eating plenty of fresh fruits, vegetables, and healthy fats like extra virgin olive oil. You still have the freedom to indulge with brain-boosting fish, heart-healthy whole grains, and seafood and sporadically can enjoy a nice steak dinner. This diet is not limiting you to be mindful of your calorie intake or not to consume other important food groups.

The recipes in this book allow you to begin trying out delicious, flavorful, and healthy Mediterranean inspired meals. You have a number of breakfasts, lunch, and dinner options that are sure to satisfy and please everyone in your home. These recipes c be your starting point in taking control of your health.

You now have a better understanding that this diet is not about just losing weight. It is not a diet that allows you to eat your weight in pasta, or drink equal amounts of red wine. It has shown that you can use food as a form of natural medicine to reduce and eliminate the risk of many serious health conditions. You have learned how your food directly affects the way your body functions and when it is deprived of the nutrients it needs it will not be able to perform appropriately.

Now that you have all this information on how you can maintain and achieve optimal health, it is up to you to decide. Will you continue to choose a life where the foods you eat leads you down a road to illness and preventable suffering? Or will you make the change now to live your life and be the healthiest and happiest version of you? All you have to do is start with one small change and then go from there. Once you begin to see the benefits from that one small choice you will be eager to try more and soon you will be living a Mediterranean lifestyle that is significantly more satisfying.

Finally, this book was intended to assist you recognize that diet does not need to make you give up some of your beloved foods. Instead, it allows you to find new favorites that will improve your overall health. Allow the food you enjoy today to be your medicine for your future.

CPSIA information can be obtained
at www.ICGtesting.com
Printed in the USA
LVHW032101060521
686681LV00015B/789